# HOW TO STAY YOUNG FOREVER

Education and tips how to feel and look younger

# Table of Contents

Escape Aging ...................................................................................1

How To Look Younger ........................................................................3

Lie Without Saying A Word ................................................................5

Places Where People Live Young In Their Old Age ..........................7

Maintaining a health Diet .................................................................10

Staying Hydrated .............................................................................12

Regular Exercise ..............................................................................13

Keep that brain working ...................................................................15

Basic Skincare .................................................................................17

A healthy home ................................................................................19

Where you live...................................................................................21

Managing stress................................................................................22

On Being YOUNG.............................................................................24

Say Hello To A Forever Young You ...................................................27

# ESCAPE AGING

What if you can escape the inescapability of time and just enjoy the pleasure of looking young? Quite difficult? Definitely not. Looking youthful and chirpy is just a matter of giving extra care for yourself and emphasizing your features, surely bringing out the best of what you got. So start defying your age now with some easy steps.

## Stopping smoking

As early as 1800's, it was already observed that smoking has detrimental effects on the skin. Two centuries later, people became more aware of this because these effects are evident among chronic smokers. Some of these consequences include premature lines and folds stemming from the corner of the eyes to the zygomatic area (in the aging process, wrinkles are a natural element , but smoking speeds this up); dry and leathery appearance of the skin; grey-pallor complexion; a haggard appearance; and some more.

These changes are brought about by the processes that a cigar's ingredients bring about to the body. Nicotine, a vasoconstrictor (one that constricts the blood vessels), inhibit the smooth and easy flow of oxygen and nutrients to their destination. Nicotine also causes a diuretic effect on the body which causes a reduction of the skin's moisture level, hereby making it tough and dry.

Carbon monoxide, a harmful component produced by smoking, has higher affinity to blood cells than oxygen. That means it reduces the amount of oxygen to many areas.

Smoking also contains a large number of free radicals that attack healthy cells and damage normal tissues.

Smoking reduces Vitamin A and collagen in the body. Vitamin A is used in the repairing function of the body. Collagen, on the other hand, is a protein that produces new and healthy skin.

## Proper posture

Sitting up straight and putting shoulders back are very important for your health and appearance. A good posture can make you look slimmer, taller, and confident. Many regard people with correct posture as young, happy, and at ease with their disposition. A good posture can even give you an instant weight loss of 10 pounds in the eyes of others. Its benefits, by the way, are not just for the outside.

A correct posture primarily puts muscles, joints, bones, and your organs to where they are supposed to sit. It reduces the risk of having back and neck problems, arthritis, and other pains. A proper one too can help prevent the spine from becoming abnormally fixed which can lead to fatigue, headaches, and some problems with organs and functioning. With a proper posture, one can also experience less strain because one wouldn't overuse his muscles.

Stretching hourly and practicing the proper posture every hour can help strengthen the muscles that will be needed to hold the body erect.

Having sex at least three times a week A 10-year study indicated that couples who are in their 40's who have sex at least three times a week look younger than those who enjoy it less often. The study even indicated that the faces of these couple have less lines and wrinkles, and have smoother and suppler skin. They credited this to the wonders of Oxytocin. It is a hormone released during sex that reduces stress. Having sex at nighttime is helpful, too!

It helps you to have a tight sleep so body is more rested. So, what are you planning to do now? Go ahead and feel young.

# HOW TO LOOK YOUNGER

The first thing you should do to look younger is to acknowledge that there are good things in store for you, and you deserve to have those. So it's all about setting your mind to get to your end. You must value the thought that almost all good things in life are brought into fruition with the right attitude and positive thinking.

So now, are you set to defy aging and look young? If you are, then these age-defying tips will surely help you look youthful easily.

**Tip 1**

No matter what you do, whether you have a demanding schedule or just being lazy in your cozy home, make sure you are getting enough sleep- and a good one at that. Your eyes will first tell if you have had enough sleep. A pair of eye-bug-free and sparkling eyes definitely makes you look younger. But how many is the suggested sleeping duration?

Perhaps you were brought up thinking that you should sleep at least 8 hours a day. Well, you should not. A new study says that those who sleep 6-7 hours live longer and healthier. Too much slumber is not good for you. In fact, sleeping for five hours is better than sleeping three hours more than that.

To have a good sleep, take some natural soporifics. These are substances that can induce sleeping. Milk is a very good example. Sex and a little aerobic may also help you sleep well.

**Tip 2**

Keep you hair short. A long hair puts in more years to your appearance, actually making you look like a tired and worn-down witch. Trying a shorter do can improve your youthfulness. Tell your hairdresser to give you side swept bangs to expose your beautiful face. Adding layers can also make our hair look lively and shinier. A little highlight may also do.

Putting on a darker hair (dark brown or black) does not only make you younger, but also coats up those grey hair.

**Tip 3**

Live in a clean environment. People who live older like the centenarians have some surrounding things in common: little stress, unpolluted air, good water, and unspoiled nature. Planting more trees in your area and planting more plants in your garden can help you provide cleaner air. More plants in the area mean more oxygen to breathe. Remember that what we breathe is the exact thing they exhale, and vice versa.

**Tip 4**

Do not put a lot of makeup. Yes, makeup can make you look pretty. But its amount, composition, and its style can make or break you. Keeping makeup light won't make you look like a villain. Use more pastel colors and those with lighter tones instead of the dark antagonistic-like colors.

Also try lipsticks with brown shade. These would make you look more natural and a lot of ears younger

**Tip 5**

Take care of your teeth. Ever notice there are a lot of old people who only have false teeth? This is because as we age, our body absorbs and stores less calcium (which also explains why old women are prone to osteoporosis).

So avoid losing your teeth permanently. Brushing every after meal is the most basic yet the most helpful habit for a good-looking set of teeth. Use teeth whitening products that can make you teeth white and shiny. Coffee and tea can stain your teeth instantly so a brush after is really helpful.

Going to the dentist at least twice a year is very important. And never forget to drink at least two glasses of milk a day, like what we teach to the real young ones.

# LIE WITHOUT SAYING A WORD

**Tips on Staying Youthful**

Stop waking up in the morning and dreading having to look in the mirror because you look "old". Instead, wake up to a relaxing full-body stretch and yawn unapologetically. Smile afterwards. If maintaining a youthful state-of-mind was as easy as that, everybody could just wake up to a good mood. Well, that can be a start. However, staying youthful means more than just those fancy chemicals advertised on TV promising you a "youthful glow" after seven days or so.

If you really want to take it seriously, first, you examine the things and the values which are attributed to being "old". Examples of such are being "no fun", "unfashionable", "irritable" and "weak". Let's dissect these attributes and turn them 180 degrees around.

## SAY YES TO FUN!

Remember when you were a teenager? When the world seemed to lack boundaries and when rules are made to be broken? Feel that rush. I am not suggesting you become a criminal. It's just that when we get older, our priorities become tweaked. Readjust them again and insert some fun into it. Eat street ice cream once again! Have a Big Mac once in a while!

Get your nails painted regularly. Hang out with your younger peers—your nieces count!—once in a while. It will keep you on your toes about what "the funnest fun" feels like. And trust me, it's a high that no other drug (or anti-aging cream) can provide.

## STAY UPDATED IN FASHION

Fashion is both an art and a discipline. However, it's not as hard as you think. There are general rules like matching your bag with your shoes, not wearing more than three colors at once, etc. There are certain fashion styles that never fade. Jeans, for example, is a worldwide classic. Learn how to use them properly. Read fashion magazines apt for your age, surf the internet for celebrity styles or even chat to your peers about it.

## TURN THAT FROWN UPSIDE DOWN

Smile! Nothing brings more negative vibes than a sulky frown. In case you haven't heard yet, it takes three times more number of facial muscles to frown than to smile. So smile! In fact, studies show that the mere act of curving your lips upward—even if you're not really smiling—releases endorphins (the get-happy hormones) throughout your body.

If you're trying to score a date, smiling will ease the tension down and makes you look more approachable. Moreover, notice the people in their 40s who always smile. They have an unexplainable, beautiful, youthful aura that works like an invisible halo that makes them always pleasing to the eye. You too, can be like them. It's all about attracting positivity in your life. Start by smiling.

GET THOSE MUSCLES MOVING

# Places Where People Live Young In Their Old Age

A long life is one of man's greatest dreams. But this dream can never be pulled off by chance. A long and healthy one starts with having good genes, but definitely, it is not your genes alone that can determine if you'll live past the 100 mark. What you take and what you do is a huge factor. But many age-conscious people in the world find very notable places where many inhabitants live long and healthy lives. What then can we learn from these distinct communities?

## Okinawa, Japan

With over a million inhabitants in this southern Japanese island, more than 900 of them have already lived more than a century. There are five more Okinawans who live to be 100 years old or so compared to other places in Japan. And the number of their centenarians is four times as many in America and in Britain.

One distinct characteristic of the Okinawans is the ability to be healthy even until their end. Researchers observed that these people tend to age slower than others. They even work as long as they can which grants these people ikigai, a sense of purpose.

Okinawans eat low-salt, low-fat, anti-oxidant rich foods such as fish, tofu, soya products, and seaweeds. A wide range of healthy foods like fruits and vegetables are also included in their rainbow diet. Not to mention, the age-defying tea is a mainstay in any meal.

But what they don't eat may also be their secret to long life. Hara hachibu is a distinct cultural practice in this place wherein they eat until they are 80% full, consuming around 1, 200 calories in a day. Why this practice makes them young is still not understood that much.

## Loma Linda, California

In this Californian city populated by the Seventh-day Adventists, citizens observe the healthy lifestyle the church promotes –having a vegetarian diet, and abstinence from smoking or drinking. That is why a lot from this city are living five or ten years longer than their neighboring areas.

That practice can well-explain that. However, scientist discovered that this practice is not done by everyone in this area, yet, they still live longer than the average.

As many claim, this community's secret is their faith. It really does raise a question if there is something about being spiritual that makes their life longer.

Researchers don't fully understand but there's this remarkable fact that makes everyone curious. It's been known for a couple of decades already that people who regularly go to the church, whatever their religion is, live more than those who don't. Some say that those who go to church on a regular basis have considerably lower levels of stress, and perhaps, because of this, these people are able to deal with stress better.

## Ovvoda, Sardinia

This small town in Italy boasts many centenarians among its 1, 700 residents. Even more notably, there are as many men who live longer as women, kicking the trend in the world. Their secret is not only the Mediterranean diet, but also their genes.

For centuries, the families in this place lived in isolation, and married only their fellow Sardinian. So, from a genetic point of view, marriage among relatives provides positive results like centenarians.

With that said, interbreeding in this place seems to have caused their people to live a longer life. This phenomenon even made some scientist discover specific genes that are associated with long life.

Oh come on! Who says you're bedridden? Get those muscles moving! Take an early morning jog and release more endorphins! Try walking to your destination if it's the sun is not so glaring. It's about time that you get out of your home and welcome the world outside!

Experts suggest backyard sports like Frisbee, badminton and table tennis. However, if you seem to not have time for these sports (say, even on weekends) try doing a fifteen minute full-body stretch right after you wake up. It gives you time to meditate and plan your day ahead. Moreover, it also improves your flexibility. Work on it so you don't have to ask someone to get the slipper stuck under the sofa again. It's not yoga, but hey, you will get there.

The best thing about this is that you don't have to eat a "special food" or buy "special equipment". You will hate having to eat oatmeal and bananas for the rest of your life and without turning your state-of-mind the way it should be, the treadmill you might purchase will just look forlorn in one corner.

Youth is all about embracing life to the fullest. You can make youth eternal. Remember, Sex and the City? Samantha was still steaming hot even when she was fifty.

# Maintaining a health Diet

While there is no magic food that can keep you young forever, a healthy diet rich in nutrients, vitamins, and antioxidants can help prevent age-related diseases and maintain a youthful appearance. Here are some particular foods that you can eat to stay young:

1. Berries: Berries such as blueberries, strawberries, and raspberries are rich in antioxidants that help protect the body from cell damage caused by free radicals. Antioxidants have been shown to slow the aging process, improve memory and reduce the risk of chronic diseases like cancer, heart disease, and diabetes.

2. Fish: Fatty fish such as salmon, trout, and sardines are rich in omega-3 fatty acids that have been shown to reduce inflammation, improve heart health, and prevent age-related cognitive decline. They also contain vitamin D that helps protect the skin from UV radiation and promote bone health.

3. Nuts: Nuts such as almonds, walnuts, and peanuts are rich in healthy fats, protein, and fiber, which can help maintain a healthy weight and reduce the risk of chronic diseases. They also contain vitamin E, which protects the skin from sun damage and improves the appearance of fine lines and wrinkles.

4. Dark Chocolate: Dark chocolate contains flavonoids that can improve heart health, lower blood pressure, and reduce the risk of chronic diseases. It also contains antioxidants that help protect the skin from free radical damage and improve blood flow, which can maintain a youthful appearance.

5. Leafy Greens: Leafy greens such as spinach, kale, and collard greens are rich in antioxidants, vitamins, and minerals such as vitamin C, vitamin K, and beta-carotene that can protect the body against cell damage

caused by free radicals. They can also reduce the risk of chronic diseases like heart disease, cancer, and diabetes.

6. Green tea: Green tea contains antioxidants that help protect the body against cell damage caused by free radicals. It also contains polyphenols that promote healthy aging, improve cognitive function and prevent age-related diseases.

7. Citrus Fruits: Citrus fruits such as oranges, lemons, and grapefruits are rich in vitamin C that promotes collagen production, which can improve skin elasticity and reduce the appearance of wrinkles.

In summary, incorporating foods that are high in antioxidants, vitamins, and minerals into your daily diet can help prevent age-related diseases, protect the body from cell damage, and maintain a youthful appearance as you age.

# Staying Hydrated

Water. Water is essential for maintaining a healthy body and skin, but there is no specific type of water that can guarantee anti-aging benefits. However, some types of water are better than others for optimal health and hydration. Here is a breakdown of some water types and their potential health benefits:

1. Filtered water: Filtered water is any water that has been purified through a filtration system to remove impurities, chemicals, and contaminants. Filtered water can help improve overall health and hydration by removing impurities and chemicals that can potentially harm the body.

2. Alkaline water: Alkaline water has a higher pH level than regular tap water, typically between 7.5 and 9.5. Some proponents of alkaline water claim that it can help neutralize the acid in the body and prevent chronic diseases, such as cancer and osteoporosis. While research is still limited, studies have shown that drinking alkaline water may help improve hydration and decrease acid reflux symptoms.

3. Mineral water: Mineral water is natural water that contains dissolved minerals and trace elements, such as magnesium and calcium. Some studies suggest that mineral water can help improve digestion, boost the immune system, and promote overall health and well-being.

4. Spring water: Spring water is sourced from natural springs and contains minerals and nutrients that may provide health benefits. In addition to being a good source of hydration, spring water may also support healthy bones and muscles, boost the immune system, and promote healthy skin. In general, drinking enough water and staying hydrated is essential for maintaining good health and promoting youthful skin. The right water for you depends on your individual needs and preferences. It is recommended that adults drink at least eight cups (64 ounces) of water per day, with additional fluids to replace lost fluids through sweating or urination.

# Regular Exercise

Exercise. Regular exercise is essential for maintaining good health and promoting longevity. Incorporating different types of exercise into your routine can help you stay young and maintain a healthy body and mind. Here are some exercise types that can help you stay young:

1. Cardiovascular Exercise: Cardiovascular exercise, also known as aerobic exercise, is any type of exercise that increases your heart rate and respiration, such as running, walking, cycling, or swimming Cardiovascular exercise helps improve cardiovascular health, lower blood pressure, burn calories, reduce stress, and improve mood.

2. Strength Training: Strength training is any type of exercise that involves using resistance, such as weights, resistance bands, or bodyweight, to build muscle strength and endurance. Strength training helps improve muscle mass, increase bone density, boost metabolism, and improve posture.

3. Flexibility and Balance Training: Flexibility and balance training, such as yoga or Pilates, helps improve flexibility, balance, and joint mobility. Flexibility exercises help improve range of motion, prevent injury, and reduce stiffness, while balance exercises help prevent falls and improve coordination.

4. High-Intensity Interval Training (HIIT): HIIT involves short bursts of intense exercise followed by periods of rest or low-intensity exercise. HIIT can increase metabolism, improve cardiovascular function, and burn calories more quickly than traditional cardiovascular exercise.

5. Mind-Body Exercise: Mind-body exercises, such as Tai Chi, Qi Gong, or meditation, help reduce stress, anxiety, and promote relaxation. Mind-body exercises help improve mental and emotional well-being, prevent cognitive decline, and promote healthy aging.

In summary, incorporating different types of exercise into your routine, such as cardiovascular exercise, strength training, flexibility and balance training, high-intensity interval training, and mind-body exercise, can help you stay young and maintain a healthy and active body and mind.

# Keep That Brain Working

Keeping your brain young is important for maintaining cognitive function and preventing age-related cognitive decline. Here are some tips on how to keep your brain young:

1. Exercise Your Brain: Regular mental exercise can help keep the brain active and improve cognitive function. Try activities such as puzzles, crossword puzzles, brain teasers, Sudoku, or learning a new language or skill.

2. Stay Socially Engaged: Staying socially engaged with friends and family can help keep the brain active and stave off loneliness and depression. Join a social club, volunteer, or attend community events.

3. Manage Stress: Chronic stress can damage the brain and accelerate cognitive decline. Find healthy ways to manage stress, such as meditation, yoga, or deep breathing exercises.

4. Get Enough Sleep: Getting sufficient sleep is essential for the body and the brain to function properly. Aim for 7-9 hours of restful sleep every night.

5. Maintain a Healthy Diet: A diet rich in nutrients such as omega-3 fatty acids, antioxidants, and vitamins can help protect the brain and improve cognitive function. Include foods such as fatty fish, nuts, fruits, and vegetables in your diet.

6. Exercise Regularly: Regular exercise can help improve blood flow to the brain and improve cognitive function. Aim for at least 150 minutes of moderate activity or 75 minutes of vigorous activity per week.

7. Stay Mentally Active: Engage in activities that challenge your mind such as reading, writing, or playing strategy games. This can help keep your brain young and prevent age-related cognitive decline.

In summary, keeping your brain young requires a mix of lifestyle changes such as regular physical and mental exercise, a healthy diet, social engagement, stress management, and good sleep hygiene. By incorporating these tips into your daily routine, you can maintain a healthy and active brain as you age.

# Basic Skincare

Skincare products There are many skincare products available on the market, and it can be overwhelming to choose the right ones for your skin. The following products are popular and have been recommended by skincare experts and users alike for their effectiveness in maintaining healthy, youthful-looking skin:

1. Cleanser: A good cleanser is essential for removing dirt, oil, and makeup from the skin. Look for a gentle cleanser that doesn't strip the skin of natural oils, and contains ingredients like salicylic acid, glycerin, or hyaluronic acid to help hydrate and exfoliate the skin.

2. Toner: Toners are used to remove any last traces of dirt or oil left on the skin and restore the skin's pH balance. Look for a toner that contains antioxidants, vitamins, and other ingredients that can help soothe and protect the skin.

3. Serum: Serums are lightweight, fast-absorbing liquids that contain high concentrations of active ingredients such as vitamin C, retinoids, or peptides. They are used to treat specific skin concerns like dark spots, fine lines, and acne.

4. Moisturizer: A moisturizer is essential for hydrating and protecting the skin. Look for a moisturizer that contains ingredients like hyaluronic acid, jojoba oil, or ceramides, that can help repair and protect the skin's barrier.

5. Sunscreen: Sunscreen protects the skin from harmful UV rays that can cause premature aging, skin damage, and cancer. Look for a broad-spectrum sunscreen with an SPF of 30 or higher, and apply it daily, even on cloudy days.

6. Face oil: Face oil can help hydrate and nourish the skin, improving its overall texture and appearance. Look for a face oil that includes

ingredients like rosehip oil, argan oil, or squalane that can help strengthen the skin barrier and reduce inflammation.

7. Retinol cream: Retinol is a form of vitamin A that is used to reduce the appearance of fine lines, wrinkles, and other signs of aging. Retinol creams should be applied at night and followed by a moisturizer and sunscreen in the morning.

In conclusion, the above wonder products for the skin can be used to build

# A HEALTHY HOME

Home. Your home is your sanctuary, and it should feel warm, inviting, and pleasant. Sweetening your home can help create a welcoming and comfortable environment that promotes relaxation and well-being. Here are some steps to sweeten your home and feel good:

1. Clean and Declutter: A clean and decluttered home can instantly make you feel better. Take the time to declutter your space and clean any dirty or messy areas. A clean and organized home can reduce stress and anxiety and promote a sense of calmness.

2. Bring in Fresh Flowers: Fresh flowers have a calming and relaxing effect on the mind and can instantly sweeten your home. Place vases of fresh flowers in various rooms to add color and fragrance to your space.

3. Add Soft Lighting: Soft lighting can create a warm and inviting atmosphere in your home. Use lamps, candles, or string lights to create a cozy, comfortable environment.

4. Use Pleasant Scents: Pleasant scents can positively impact your mood and promote relaxation. Use essential oils, candles, or air fresheners with scents like lavender or vanilla to create a relaxing and inviting atmosphere.

5. Hang Artwork or Photos: Hang artwork or photos that make you happy and reflect your personality. This can add visual interest to your space and make it feel more personalized and welcoming.

6. Create Comfortable Seating: Comfortable seating can make your home feel more welcoming and inviting. Invest in comfortable furniture, such as a cozy sofa or comfortable armchair, to create a comfortable and inviting space.

7. Play Music: Play soft and calming music to create a soothing and relaxing atmosphere in your home. Music can reduce stress and anxiety and promote relaxation and well-being.

In summary, sweetening your home can help create a more comfortable and welcoming environment that promotes relaxation and well-being. By following the above steps, you can create a relaxing and inviting interior that you and your loved ones will enjoy spending time in.

# Where You Live

People live There are several places in the world where people live younger in their old age. These regions are called "blue zones," named after the blue ink that was used to circle them on a map. Here are some of the most well-known blue zones:

1. Nicoya Peninsula, Costa Rica: People in Nicoya Peninsula have a higher life expectancy than the rest of Costa Rica and are known for their active and social lifestyle. They follow the traditional "Mesoamerican diet" that is low in calories but high in nutrients.

2. Sardinia, Italy: Sardinian diet is mostly plant-based and includes whole grains, beans, fruits, and vegetables. The people in Sardinia are also known for their strong community ties and social support systems.

3. Okinawa, Japan: People in Okinawa have lower rates of chronic diseases and higher life expectancy. They follow a traditional, plant-based diet with a focus on nutrition and balanced meals. The Okinawan people are also known for their strong social support networks and active lifestyle.

4. Ikaria, Greece: People in Ikaria live long and healthy lives, and they have a strong sense of purpose and sense of community. They follow a traditional Mediterranean diet that is rich in plants, beans, and whole grains and includes regular physical activity and stress reduction practices.

5. Loma Linda, California: In Loma Linda, a large population of Seventh-day Adventists have lower rates of chronic diseases and higher life expectancy. They follow a vegetarian diet with an emphasis on whole grains and legumes and engage in regular physical activity and stress reduction practices.

In summary, "blue zones" are areas around the world where people tend to live longer and healthier lives due to their lifestyle habits and social support systems. These habits include a plant-based diet, regular physical activity, and a strong sense of community and purpose.

# Managing Stress

Stress management is vital for maintaining good physical and mental health, as well as staying young. Modern-day lifestyle is replete with uncertainties that make stress management imperative. The process of stress management involves identifying stressors and finding effective ways to deal with them. The following essay elucidates the practical ways of managing stress and staying young.

One of the most effective ways of managing stress is through regular exercise. Exercise is not only beneficial for the body but also the mind. It helps in reducing stress levels by releasing endorphins (feel-good hormones) in the body. Endorphins have a calming effect on the mind and reduce stress. Regular exercise also strengthens the immune system, improves blood circulation, and helps maintain a healthy weight, which is essential in staying young.

Another way of reducing stress levels is through relaxation techniques such as meditation, deep breathing, and yoga. Meditation and deep breathing help in calming the mind and reducing anxiety levels. Yoga is a gentle form of exercise that combines both relaxation techniques and exercise, and it has been shown to be an effective way of managing stress.

Eating a healthy diet is another way of managing stress and staying young. Eating a balanced diet that is rich in fruits, vegetables, whole grains, proteins, and healthy fats helps in providing the nutrients essential for the body to function correctly. It also helps in maintaining a healthy weight and reducing the risk of chronic diseases.

Getting enough sleep is crucial in managing stress and staying young. Lack of sleep has been linked to high-stress levels and several health conditions such as obesity, diabetes, and cardiovascular disease. It is recommended that adults get seven to nine hours of sleep per night to help manage stress levels and maintain overall health.

In conclusion, stress management is essential for maintaining good physical and mental health and staying young. Regular exercise, relaxation techniques, eating a healthy diet, and getting enough sleep are practical ways of managing stress. Incorporating these practices into daily life will go a long way in promoting health and wellness.

# On Being Young

One can never stop the passing of time. Hence, aging is inevitable. But being and looking old now seems to be just an option. One can still havethe better option, and that is to feel and look young. But what does thisideal really mean? Is it limited to a radiant skin and wrinkle-free skin?Is it just the absence of the torment of arthritis?

Definitely not. Staying young encompasses a wide range of ideas and includes more good conditions than the aforementioned. Being young comes from the mind, body, and the heart.

**Being sharp**

As people age, they tend to be less smart, alert, and intelligent. Compared to a young grade-schooler, an old person can hardly recite the multiplication table with ease, speed, and accuracy. This is because as they age, neurons weaken and lessens its ability to recall facts and details. To avoid this and be young in the mental capacity, people should do few good things.

Meditating, resting well, and getting enough sleep help brain to be at ease. Playing board games like chess, scrabbles, and word factory can help boost your brain. Eating a healthy diet with less cholesterol is helpful.

Doing moderate aerobic exercises can produce Brain-Derived Neurotrohic Factor (BDNF) that maintains a healthy neuron. BDNF is a protein that acts on certain neurons of the central nervous system (CNS) and the peripheral nervous system (PNS) that aids in the survival of existing neurons. Adding to that, BDNF encourages the growth and differentiation of new neurons and synapses.

**Being healthy**

Being young is almost synonymous to being healthy. If one is at his optimum health, he is sure to look and feel good, which is by the way, how many define being young. As we all know, to be healthy is to guard your own body. Eat more nutrient-packed greens, more Omega-3 containingfish, and other healthy stuff like whole-grains, tomatoes, milk, fruits,and water.

And of course, less foods containing tons of cholesterol (burger patties,barbecues, fries) and sodium (chips, MSG, salt). Exercising for at leastten minutes a day, avoiding stress, and a regular visit to a doctor are of great help to staying healthy.

Being young wouldn't be complete without a healthy skin. As the body's largest organ, it can tell how well your health is and how well you are aging. Eating at least 5 serving of anti-oxidant rich fruits and vegetables, sipping anti-oxidant rich green tea, and drinking at least 8glasses of pure water a day are of prime necessity.

Not to mention, a smile can really deceive others of your age.

## Being optimistic and vigorous

Having an encouraging, dynamic, and balanced approach or outlook towardsyour individual and collective possibilities is a healthy advantage. Notonly does it provide you with better results in what you seek, it also gives your youthful energy a boost.

Optimism and vigor shape a huge part in the expansion of your emotionallife. If you wish to live well and young, you will have to remove the self-defeating pessimism from your mind, and replace with a constructive attitude.

Being young is also being optimistic and vigorous, and that requires moreof us than exhibiting a compelled smile and telling yourself, "you can doit." Being young is living your life at full capacity, and we can only go beyond what we think we can if we expand ourselves rather than holding yourself back, and rather than putting you forward. After all, who got blinded by looking at the brighter side of life?

Indeed, being young is also skin-deep. And because it is, you should examine a little more within you to know whether you too can feel andlook young. And if you will, the inside will radiate a more beautifulbeing.

# Say Hello To A Forever Young You

As you grow older, your priorities become redirected. Before, the greatest problem you could possibly have is what to wear on your school/office wash day. Fast forward, the hurdle you're facing is a 2-year old child. Fast forward again, you look in the mirror and realize that all those worrying and "problematizing" finally took their toll on your skin.

It's about time that you know yourself more and pay less attention to your outside appearance. After all, what really matters is how you feel inside. A rich man can feel that he still needs to get richer; so in principle, he is not rich at all. However, a poor man can be more contented than a millionaire and at the end of the day, the poor man becomes happier. Let's cruise through what keeps one young by not applying a wonder cream or doing a wonder work-out.

## MEDITATE

The day-in, day-out stress will make you feel like "slipping away" from the things which used to make you happy and things which used to make you feel like a child again. Rekindle these good memories by meditating at least ten minutes a day. Take some time to detach yourself from the world and think. You don't need to philosophize deeply or to draft your next blog entry. Just enjoy some silence and a piece of world peace.

Choose a ten- to fifteen-minute break in your day. Just a short while. You have twenty four hours a day. Surely you can find or MAKE time for some productive self-healing.

## KEEP A DIARY

A diary is a very important tool for a writer. However, even if you're not a writer or even if you are not a grammar expert, it is also advisable to keep a diary. A diary is an outlet. It is a friend which will listen, will not judge and handy also. A diary is a tool of letting- go of the bad things that have happened to you which pull you back from moving forward.

You need to pass on some of your worries somewhere so you can focus to more important things like the relationships around you and the smallestget-happy detail of your everyday life. Keeping a diary also is like keeping a record of your psychological states. There are people who freakout when they realize that they're starting to age and surely you don't want to be one of them.

Don't look at it as a task. Just write whenever you want to. Even in themiddle of the night. Isn't it just neat that someone will listen to everydetail of your nightmare and not brand you a lunatic?

## HAVE A DATE WITH YOURSELF

The most important person in your life should still be yourself EVEN IF you have aged. Remember when you were younger, when all you wanted was the latest gadget and the in pair of jeans? That's exactly how you should still feel, albeit being more mature. Try not going into the selfishpath; that's too much.

Watch a movie alone; save yourself from the pains of having to explain tosomeone how the plot should have gone. Devour your favorite cake alone, go shoe-shopping alone, brim in front of the mirror and say "I'm the king/queen of the world"! Err, please remember to do the last thing alone too. Please. It's for your own good.

When you were young, it was all about you. Now that you're older, let itstill be all about you. The secret to staying young is all in the mind. You don't even need to get out of your home right? There's no use studying what certain chemicals can do to save your skin while not learning to know, love and embrace your self. Your beautiful, ethereal self.